My Knee Hurts!

Handbook for Seniors with Knee Pain

D1636859

by Orthopaedic Surgeons

James D. Hundley, M.D. and Richard J. Nasca, M.D.

MyBones Series Book #3
MyBones Publishing Company
September 2018

Previous Books in the MyBones Series

My Hip Hurts!
Causes and Treatments of Hip Pain in Seniors
2018

My Back Hurts!
Handbook for Seniors with Back Pain
2018

Upcoming Books in the MyBones Series

My Neck Hurts!
Handbook for Seniors with Neck Pain

My Shoulder Hurts!
My Elbow Hurts!
Handbook for Seniors with Shoulder or Elbow Pain

Introduction

This is the third in our **MyBones** series of condition-specific books for non-physicians. Each book focuses on specific areas: neck, back, hip, knee, shoulder, elbow, hand, ankle and foot, along with several other topics. Please search on Amazon from time to time to see if a **MyBones** book addressing your area of concern has become available.

Medical science is complicated. Physicians necessarily use language uncommon to most people, even those highly educated in other disciplines. Thoughtful people wish to understand their medical problems. We intend for this book to provide you and your loved ones with a better understanding of your diagnosis and options for treatment.

In this book, two seasoned orthopaedic surgeons combine over 100 years of training and experience to help demystify the language of our profession. Moreover, we offer opinions on how we believe our loved ones and ourselves should be treated.

This information should help you better communicate with your physician, as well as provide relevant questions to get useful answers. We want you to avoid problems when possible and take an active role in helping your surgeon determine the best course to follow when help is needed.

To become orthopaedic surgeons, we graduated from medical school and followed with five years of specialized training in orthopaedic surgery under intense supervision. Then we passed an arduous board examination in our specialty. After two years in the U.S. Navy, Dr. Nasca went into academic surgery where he practiced orthopaedic surgery and trained future surgeons. After two years as an orthopaedic surgeon in the U.S. Air Force, Dr. Hundley joined a group of orthopaedic surgeons in private practice.

We take responsibility for what we say, but please remember that we are expressing our opinions based on training and experience. Medical science changes rapidly, so what seems to be true today may not seem so tomorrow. Furthermore, it is common for medical people to have different opinions, so it should not surprise you if your surgeon has opinions different from ours. We are telling you what we think and believe to be true, but there are many ways to assess and approach difficult problems.

Reading this book does not make one an expert. It cannot replace professional, in-person consultation. If your condition is persistent or worsening or you need more information about your particular case, please see an orthopaedic surgeon as soon as possible.

Above all, we offer this book as a basis for an informed discussion with your physician. If it provides a level of understanding that can improve your outcome, we have accomplished our goal.

Be enlightened! Be empowered! Be healthy!

Table of Contents and Overview

Introduction

Chapter 1: Dave's Knee
The saga of Dave's knee from injury to knee replacement, reflecting the evolution of orthopaedic surgery over the past 50 years

Chapter 2: Description of the Knee Joint
The knee is a complex joint held in place by ligaments and powered and stabilized by muscles. The menisci provide additional stability and cushioning. The kneecap provides leverage to assist in straightening the knee.

Chapter 3: Causes of Knee Pain
Torn menisci and ligaments, arthritis, and tendonitis are common causes of knee pain; cancer and infection are less common. Pain can be referred from the hip and spine or originate from poor circulation.

Chapter 4: History, Physical Examination, and Laboratory Studies
When you see your surgeon, you will be asked what bothers you most about your knee. Then you will be asked a series of questions designed to give the surgeon specific information useful in diagnosis. An examination of your knee will be performed. Imaging studies (X-Rays, MRI, CT scans, and bone scans) and blood tests are invaluable in further evaluating disorders and making treatment recommendations.

Chapter 5: Treatment of Knee Pain
Medications, injections, physical therapy and the benefits of compression sleeves, braces, and walking aids are discussed.

Total joint replacement is the most likely procedure for advanced arthritis of the knee. Arthroscopic surgery has a role but one that is more limited in seniors than in the younger population. Some other procedures are briefly discussed, but total knee replacement is the likely choice.

Chapter 6: Potential Complications of Knee Surgery
Even the healthiest of patients having surgery that was done extremely well are subject to experiencing complications. The presence of comorbidities such as diabetes, vascular disease, pulmonary disease, immune deficiencies, and obesity increase the risk of complications. This chapter discusses potential complications, but the chances of suffering any are below 5%.

Glossary
Medical terms and phrases are defined to help readers better understand the problems and treatments are described.

Acknowledgements
We express appreciation to those who have inspired and helped us.

About the Authors
Brief biographies of the authors are provided.

Reviewer Comments
Commentaries by readers are shared.

Chapter 1: Dave's Knee

Dave was not a gifted athlete, but he enjoyed high school basketball and football. He continued recreational sports in college but twisted his knee playing intramural basketball. After that, it was never the same. The orthopaedic surgeon recommended "living with it", which he did for several years. Later, Dave's knee not only began to "give way", but it would frequently "lock" such that he could not straighten it or walk until it "unlocked". Something needed to be done.

An arthrogram (x-ray taken after injecting "dye" into the joint) confirmed a torn medial meniscus. Since arthroscopic surgery had not been invented, "open" surgery to remove the torn meniscus was performed through a six-inch incision. He was told that the meniscus that had often jammed between the bones had damaged the joint surfaces. After a few weeks he was much better, but his knee swelled and hurt with jogging and long walking.

Twenty years later it had worsened causing Dave pain and giving way. MRI and arthroscopic surgery had been invented, and he was diagnosed as having a lateral meniscus tear. Arthroscopic lateral menisectomy (removal of the lateral meniscus) was performed. Again, his knee was improved, but it was far from normal.

Over the years, his knee began to bow outward, and the pain increased. With prolonged standing, it cracked loud enough for others to hear. X-rays demonstrated "bone-on-bone" and a "total knee replacement" was performed. He recovered well and worked hard to regain strength and range of motion. Now he can walk unlimited distances without pain. He plays golf with no difficulty. Preferring to not wear out his artificial parts too quickly, he does not play tennis.

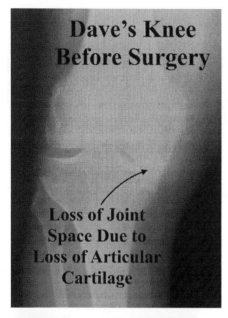

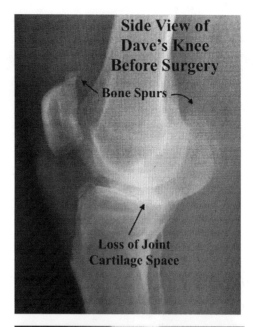

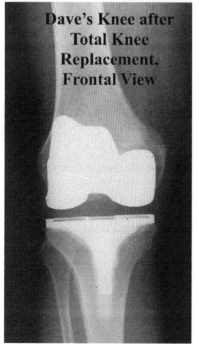

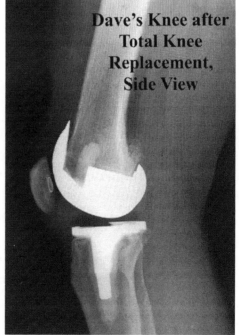

Chapter 2
Anatomy of the Knee Joint

Like most joints, the knee is an assembly of hard tissues transitioning into softer ones. The hard tissues are the bones: the femur, tibia, and patella. The parts that rub together in the joint are covered with a slightly softer, rubbery tissue called the articular cartilage. Surrounding the joint is a tough, fibrous capsule that holds everything together. Ligaments reinforce the capsule. Lining the joint is the synovial membrane, which is normally very thin and produces the oily joint fluid. The menisci are roughly half-moon-shaped structures that add cushioning and stability.

The knee is a complex hinge joint. The axis of motion changes with flexion (bending) and extension (straightening). The ends of the femur and tibia and the back of the patella are covered with "articular cartilage". It is a smooth, rubbery material that cushions and, with the aid of joint fluid, makes the ends of the bones so slick that they glide upon each other with very little friction. It has been said that the surfaces of normal joints lubricated by the oily synovial fluid are more slippery than ice on ice.

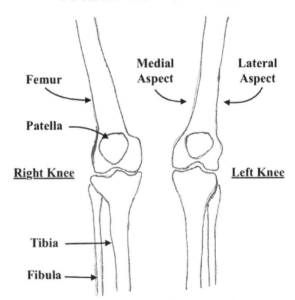

Frontal View of Knees

Femur

Medial Aspect

Lateral Aspect

Patella

Right Knee

Left Knee

Tibia

Fibula

Between the large bones of the knee (femur and tibia) are the menisci that fill spaces in the joint. When normal, they add cushioning and stability. When torn, whether through injury or fraying through years of use, they cause problems.

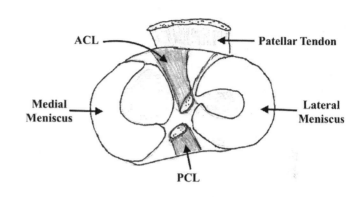

Cross-section of Knee Viewed from Above

ACL — Patellar Tendon — Medial Meniscus — Lateral Meniscus — PCL

Ligaments hold the bones together. The ones on the sides are called "collateral ligaments", one being medial (on the side toward the other knee) and the other lateral (on the side away from the other knee). They prevent the bones from rocking back and forth from side to side. In the center are the anterior cruciate (ACL) and posterior cruciate ligaments (PCL) that prevent the tibia from sliding forward and backward on the femur.

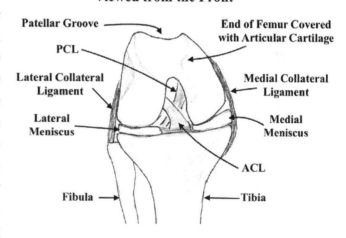

Inside of the Right Knee Viewed from the Front

Patellar Groove — PCL — Lateral Collateral Ligament — Lateral Meniscus — Fibula — End of Femur Covered with Articular Cartilage — Medial Collateral Ligament — Medial Meniscus — ACL — Tibia

Actually, there are two articulations (places where bones rub together) in the knee. The one between the femur and the tibia is dominant, but the one between the patella and the femur is important, too.

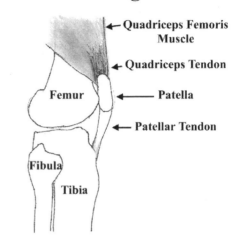

Side View of Right Knee

Quadriceps Femoris Muscle

Quadriceps Tendon

Femur

Patella

Patellar Tendon

Fibula

Tibia

The kneecap (patella) arises from within the tendon of the quadriceps muscle and physically connects to other bones only through the quadriceps and the patellar tendons. It provides leverage to the muscle to improve its efficiency in straightening the knee. As it "floats" in the muscles on the front of the knee, its position depends on a groove in the femur as well as the muscle. The backside of the patella and the femoral groove in which it resides are also covered with articular cartilage, which is subject to wear and tear.

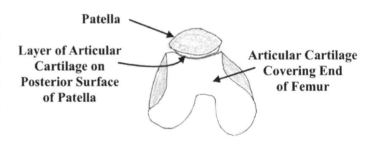

Patella

Layer of Articular Cartilage on Posterior Surface of Patella

Articular Cartilage Covering End of Femur

Cross-section View of Patella in Groove of Anterior Femur

The dominant muscles controlling the knee are the quadriceps femoris ("quads") and the hamstrings. The quads arise from the pelvis near the hip joint and the femur, creating a stabilizing half-sleeve over the front of the knee, and attach to the front of the tibia just below the knee joint. The hamstrings arise from the bottom of the pelvis behind the femur and attach to the tibia below the knee. The quads extend (straighten) the knee and hold it straight while standing and walking. A strong quad is needed to stand from a sitting position. The hamstrings bend the knee and also prevent it from uncontrolled, potentially damaging straightening when walking and running.

Chapter 3
Common Causes of Knee Pain in Seniors

Arthritis

Articular cartilage is a critical but vulnerable joint structure. It is somewhat rubbery and very slippery. It is a living substance but the cartilage cells are sparse and do not regenerate well. Once damaged, it does not repair itself. It is only a couple of millimeters thick, so you cannot lose much before the surface of the bone is exposed. Once bone is exposed, you have a badly arthritic knee. On x-ray you see a loss of the joint cartilage space, which leads to the "bone-on-bone" description you often hear about in people undergoing joint replacement. This is commonly due to "degenerative arthritis".

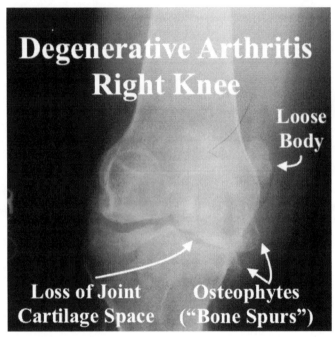

You can develop degenerative arthritis from excessive use such as a long history of running for exercise, injury, infection, obesity, and malalignment, all of which can damage the articular cartilage. The effect of most of these is self-evident, but malalignment needs some explanation. Normal human knee joints have a few degrees of valgus ("knock-kneed") alignment. If your knees are truly straight, when viewed from the front or back, they appear to be bowed outward. If your knee joint is excessively bowed outward (varus alignment) or bowed inward

Alignment
Frontal View of the Right Knee

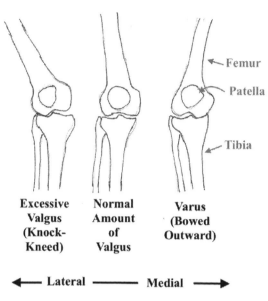

Excessive Valgus (Knock-Kneed) Normal Amount of Valgus Varus (Bowed Outward)

← Lateral ——— Medial →

(valgus alignment), excessive pressure is applied to one side of the joint or the other, ultimately resulting in degenerative arthritis.

There are two articulations (places where bones rub together) in the knee. One is between the femur and tibia; the other is between the femur and the patella (kneecap). The patella arises from within the large tendon of the quadriceps muscle and glides back and forth in a groove on the front of the end of the femur.

Sometimes the groove is too shallow, the quadriceps muscle is weak, or the angle of alignment between the femur and tibia is too great or too small. Sometimes the patella is congenitally too high or too low. Sometimes the patella is injured such as when people run into hard objects like walls or goalposts or fall onto a flexed knee. A visible fracture is not required to injure the joint between the femur and patella (patello-femoral joint). A long-ago injury as a youth can initiate deterioration that results in arthritis in the patella-femoral joint in adulthood.

Whatever the cause, the symptoms of patello-femoral arthritis are pain in the front of the knee, weakness due to pain causing one to give in to the pain when walking up or down stairs, and grinding in the front of the knee that you can feel and often hear.

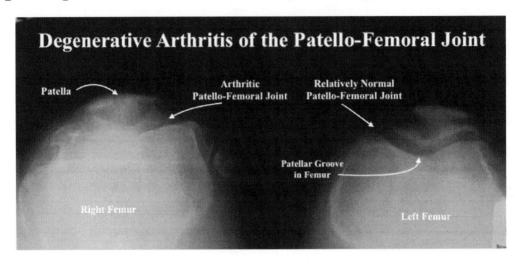

Osteoarthritis is a generalized disorder, but in an individual joint it is hard to distinguish from degenerative arthritis. In both cases, osteophytes (bone spurs) form and there is loss of articular cartilage. On x-rays, this appears as a reduction in thickness of the joint cartilage space (an apparent space between bones).

Autoimmune diseases (such as rheumatoid arthritis, systemic lupus erythematosis, and Reiter's Syndrome) are called inflammatory arthritis because they cause a reaction in the lining of the joint (the synovium) that damages articular cartilage. As opposed to osteoarthritis and degenerative arthritis, there is thinning of the bone, not thickening. The loss of articular cartilage, however, is paramount and results in bone rubbing on bone.

Gouty arthritis is also an inflammatory arthritis that causes severe, episodic pain and damage to the articular cartilage. The joint can swell and one can see redness and feel increased temperature in the skin. Gout is a metabolic disorder that can generally be controlled with diet and medications. Gouty arthritis attacks are caused by deposition of uric acid crystals in the synovial lining of the joint and often follow injury, eating certain foods, and drinking red wine. A condition called "pseudogout" is due to the deposition of a different kind of crystals. Testing the fluid in the knee is required to determine the type of gout and to be sure there is no infection.

Internal Derangement

<u>Meniscus tears</u>: With age and use, knee joints develop problems such as degenerative tears in the menisci and loose bodies. Meniscal tears can result in parts of the meniscus flipping in and out of their normal positions, sometimes getting jammed in between the bones. This can cause locking, where the knee cannot be fully straightened, and "giving way", where the knee buckles unexpectedly when walking.

In younger people, tears of menisci usually occur with athletic activities. In our senior group, they can also be the result of previous injuries. We have seen many cases of torn menisci in older people that showed evidence of old and new

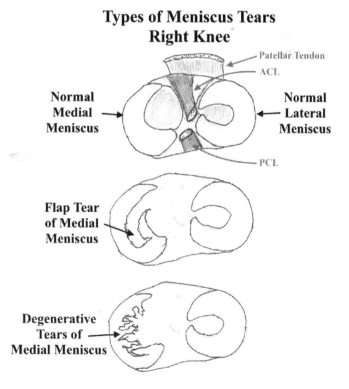

Types of Meniscus Tears
Right Knee

Patellar Tendon
ACL
Normal Medial Meniscus
Normal Lateral Meniscus
PCL
Flap Tear of Medial Meniscus
Degenerative Tears of Medial Meniscus

tears. Some had been diagnosed as having meniscal tears when young, but the symptoms subsided allowing them to erroneously assume it had "healed". Years later, the tear enlarged and the symptoms returned. Menisci become brittle with age and fray and tear more easily.

Loose bodies: Relatively minor injuries can cause bits of articular cartilage to break away from their attachment to bone. Since joint fluid nourishes articular cartilage, these small fragments grow over time, sometimes getting as large as a bird egg. They can be inconsequential, but when they get caught between the ends of the bones, they cause locking and giving way.

Ligament Injuries
The ligament injuries we usually hear about are the ACL (anterior cruciate ligament) and MCL (medial collateral ligament). Unless we are elite athletes, repair of these ligaments in seniors is usually unnecessary. As joints stiffen with age, loss of stability from tears of these ligaments is not usually problematic.

In the case of the ACL, however, fragments can flip between the joint surfaces, resulting in symptoms of locking and popping. If this persists, removal of the torn fragments may be necessary.

Tendonitis
Tendonitis results from micro tears with resultant inflammation of tendons, the tough fibrous tissue that attaches muscle to bone. The most common in the knee is patellar tendonitis, also known as "jumper's knee". Few seniors do a lot of jumping, but it can happen. More likely in seniors is that pain in the area of the patellar tendon is a result of arthritis in the patello-femoral joint.

Bursitis

Most joints have bursae that reduce friction. They allow tendons to move back and forth over bony prominences without pain. The knee has many, but the one that causes the most trouble is just below the joint on the medial side. Named the "pes anserine bursa" for the metaphorical "crow's foot" convergence of tendons that come together at this site, it can become quite painful.

Baker's Cyst / Popliteal Cyst

Richard, a 66-year-old man had been an active surfer, swimmer, biker and exercise walker for as long as he could remember. He was in excellent physical condition and could have passed for being under 50. Without injury or other obvious reason, he experienced several weeks of pain and swelling in his knee. His examination was suggestive of a tear of the medial meniscus, but his symptoms were not terrible. He embraced the option to wait and see if his symptoms would subside.

Ten days later, Richard started having pain and swelling in his calf and some in his ankle. Examination at that time revealed a small amount of fluid in his knee and tenderness over the area of his medial meniscus. He had no tenderness in the back of the knee but definitely had tenderness in the deep calf area of that leg. He had slight swelling in his ankle.

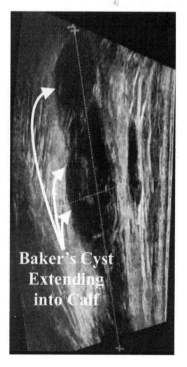

Baker's Cyst Extending into Calf

As DVT (deep vein thrombosis, also known as "blood clots" in the veins of the legs) is hard to diagnosis and can be dangerous (Please see "Chapter 5: Complications".), so an ultrasound was performed. Fortunately, he had no evidence of DVT but was found to have a large "Baker's Cyst" in his calf. Now what?

Twenty per cent of people are born with a channel connecting the interior of the knee joint to a bursa in the back of the knee. When they have a derangement in their knees causing fluid to build up under pressure inside the joint, they can get swelling in the back of the knee (an area known as the popliteal fossa). It is often called a "Baker's Cyst". If the "cyst" expands down the leg between the bone and calf muscles, it is hard to distinguish from DVT (deep vein thrombosis). You will need MRI or ultrasound to distinguish them. The cyst is not dangerous, but DVT is!

Bone Fractures About the Knee

Fractures of the hip, which are fractures of the upper femur, in seniors are relatively common and can be very debilitating. You do not often hear about fractures of the knee area, but they can be debilitating, too. These are fractures that occur in the lower end of the femur, the upper end of the tibia, and in the patella.

Fractures of the shaft of the femur, the long part between the hip and knee, can occur from falls, especially in those with low bone mass such as osteoporosis. These are commonly treated with a rod or plate that stabilizes the bone until it heals. Femur fractures that involve the knee joint usually result from high impact trauma, such as in motor vehicle crashes. The bones are broken into multiple pieces and need to be restored to as near normal as feasible. That typically involves surgery and a significant rehabilitation period.

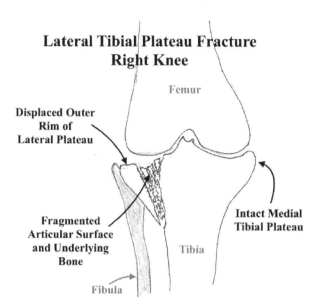

Lateral Tibial Plateau Fracture Right Knee

Femur

Displaced Outer Rim of Lateral Plateau

Fragmented Articular Surface and Underlying Bone

Intact Medial Tibial Plateau

Tibia

Fibula

More common in seniors are fractures of the upper tibia where it comprises the lower half of the knee joint. Stepping down from a chair or cabinet or a fall can produce fractures of the "tibial plateau". Since they involve the joint surface, if displaced, they need to be surgically restored to as near normal as possible. Even with an excellent repair, degenerative arthritis will likely occur. Although perfect joint restoration is usually not possible, putting the major parts of the bone back into as near normal as possible makes joint replacement in the future more feasible, so surgical treatment may be recommended.

Fractures of the smaller bone, the fibula, near the knee and down to the

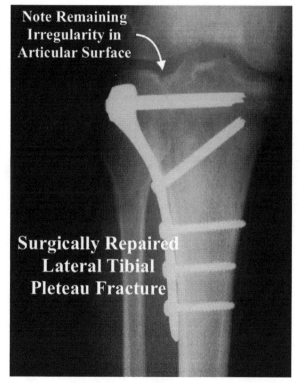

Note Remaining Irregularity in Articular Surface

Surgically Repaired Lateral Tibial Pleteau Fracture

mid-portion of the fibula, are generally of little consequence. They are treated with management of pain and swelling.

The patella is part of the extensor mechanism complex, making the quadriceps muscles more efficient. If the patellar fragments are only minimally separated, a fracture can probably be treated non-operatively by protecting it from high tension on the quadriceps until the bones unite. Even so, damage to the joint surface increases the likelihood of future arthritis between the patella and femur.

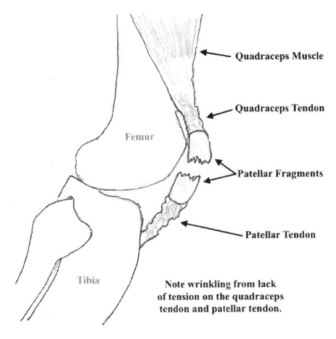

**Fracture of the Right Patella
with Disruption of the Extensor Mechanism**

Quadraceps Muscle

Quadraceps Tendon

Femur

Patellar Fragments

Patellar Tendon

Tibia

Note wrinkling from lack
of tension on the quadraceps
tendon and patellar tendon.

If the fragments are widely separated, that indicates a disruption of the extensors, which results in a disruption of the ability to actively extend the knee and hold it straight. You will not be able to walk or stand from a sitting position. Surgical fixation is usually necessary.

In cases of fractures about joints, including the knee, beginning movement of the joint as soon as possible is advised. Otherwise scar tissue will bind the joint ends together and severely compromise the desired result.

Infection

Bacterial and other infections in the knee are uncommon in seniors unless they contain foreign bodies such as artificial joints or internal fixation devices like pins or plates, or that have had penetrating injuries. The signs and symptoms are like infections elsewhere: fever, pain, redness, and swelling.

Cancer

Primary bone cancer (cancer originating in bone) is uncommon in seniors. Metastatic cancer (cancer originating elsewhere and spreading to bone) is more likely. It is also uncommon for metastatic cancer to land below the knee. That is not to say it could not happen; it is just not common.

Referred Pain to the Knee

Not all pain sensed in the knee comes from the knee itself. Hip joint mediated pain is notorious for being felt in the knee area. Hip joint pain is usually in the groin, not the buttocks, which many consider their "hip". Sometimes, rather than hurting in their groin, people will feel pain from their hip in the front of the thigh down to and including the knee.

Back pain from inflamed or compressed spinal nerves is often referred to the lower extremities. Depending on which nerves are involved, this can be in the front or back of the thigh or leg.

Arterial disease can generate pain in the legs. "Claudication", pain in the calf or behind the knee that occurs with walking, is a well-known condition caused by peripheral arterial disease (PAD, clogging of the arteries with diminished blood flow).

Chapter 4
History and Physical Examination of the Knee
Laboratory Studies

What should you expect when you visit your surgeon? Typically, he will ask you to tell him what is bothering you, and he will likely ask pesky questions so as to convert lay terms into medical ones to help define the problem. For example, if you say that your knee hurts on the inside, do you mean it is in the depths of the knee or on the medial side? That is important.

The History

Your physician needs to know specifically where it hurts and when it started. Do certain activities make it hurt? What are they? Does your pain continue after you stop that activity? How long does it continue? Can you make it stop hurting? How? Does it hurt at night? Does it wake you at night, or do you wake for other reasons and feel it? Does it lock so you cannot straighten your knee? If so, does it unlock on its own, or is there something you can do to "unlock" it? Does it "give way" and throw you off balance? Does it swell? If so, where? Does it get red and hot? Do any other joints hurt? Have you had surgery on this or the other knee? Does your back hurt? Do you hurt in the hip or the groin? Do you hurt in the calf or back of the knee when walking?

You can help your physician define your problems by considering these questions before your consultation visit. Write them and other pertinent symptoms down, so you will not get flustered and forget important information.

Be honest and forthcoming. Hiding symptoms from your physician is not in your best interests.

The Focused Physical Examination

A total body examination is not needed, so even though some body areas other than the knee will be examined, it is called a "focused" examination.

Gait: You will be observed for a limp. Your surgeon is trained to differentiate among different types of limps, which give clues to the cause of the limp and the severity of the problem.

Alignment: While standing, you will be observed to see if your knees are excessively bowed outward or bent inward.

Signs of inflammation: Does the knee appear red or feel warmer than your skin elsewhere?

Swelling: Is there swelling around the knee (edema) or is the excess fluid inside the knee joint (effusion)? Your surgeon can generally distinguish one from the other.

Tenderness: Pain is a symptom described by the patient in the history. Tenderness is determined by a painful reaction to pressure being applied to a sensitive area. The knee will be touched and pressed in several areas, with particular attention to areas that are painful.

Range of Motion: The knee should extend a few degrees beyond straight and bend (flex) to or greater than 135°. This may be estimated or measured with a goniometer (a joint range of motion measuring device).

Stability: The resistance of your knee to medial or lateral angulation with the knee fully straight and with it flexed about 20° help determine the integrity of the medial and lateral collateral ligaments. "Drawer tests" are so named because the examiner pulls the tibia forward relative to the femur when performing an anterior drawer test (like pulling open a cabinet drawer) and pushing the drawer back into the cabinet for the posterior drawer test. The anterior and the posterior drawer tests are performed with the knee flexed 90° as well as 20° to determine the integrity of the ACL and PCL. A ruptured ACL allows too much forward motion of the tibia, and a ruptured PCL allows too much backward motion.

Crepitus: Is there a sound or sensation of grinding when the knee is flexed or extended? The examiner tries to determine whether the crepitus is coming from the joint between the femur and tibia, or the femur and patella?

Meniscus Test (McMurray's Test): With the patient lying supine, the knee will be flexed as much as comfortably possible and then the leg is internally rotated. With the leg held in that position, the knee will be straightened. If the surgeon feels a "popping sensation", he is finding evidence of a meniscus tear. By doing the test with a hand on the knee, the examiner can often tell from which side (medial or lateral) the popping occurs. The maneuver is repeated with the leg in external rotation.

Hip Range of Motion: Since it is common for hip pain to be referred to the knee, the hips are examined to be certain that they move normally and without pain. If moving a hip causes the knee on the same side to hurt, the hip needs further evaluation.

Circulation: Examination of the lower extremities is incomplete until one has checked the circulation status. The examiner will feel for the posterior tibial artery pulse behind the medial aspect of the ankle and the dorsalis pedis artery pulse in the middle of the top of the foot. He can also look to see if the toenail beds are pink, and how quickly color returns after squeezing the toes to turn the nail beds white, and then removing the pressure.

Foot Examination: Looking at the feet is done to be sure there is no infection or major deformity. Severe flat footedness, for example, increases load bearing on the lateral side of the knee.

Laboratory Studies

Imaging Studies
X-rays are more useful with the patient standing since they are more likely to show narrowing of the joint space, which is an indication of loss of articular cartilage. Front and side views are obtained with the patient standing and the knees flexed about 25°. A "skyline" view is taken to show how the patella sits in its groove in the femur, and another view is taken with the knee in 60° of flexion to see if there are loose bodies hidden behind the femur.

To perform an arthrogram, your physician injects a "radiopaque" dye (one that shows up on x-ray) into the knee joint, and then takes x-rays or a CT scan to determine if there is a meniscus tear. As this test has been replaced by the MRI scan, it is rarely done today.

MRI is the best test to show meniscus tears, ligament disruptions "bone bruises", stress fractures, tumors and other abnormalities not seen or definable by x-ray. On the below MRIs, you can see structures like the menisci and articular cartilage, and you can also see that there is not really a space between the bones. The "joint cartilage space" is actually filled by articular cartilage that is not visible on x-ray.

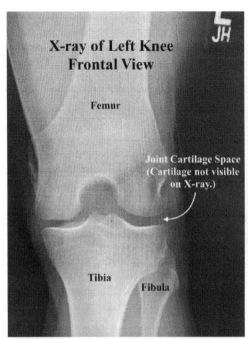

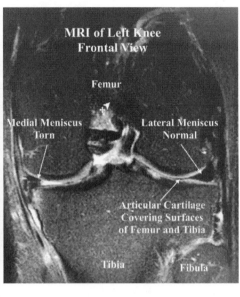

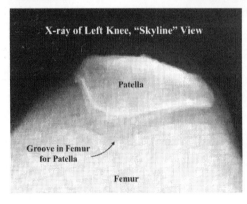

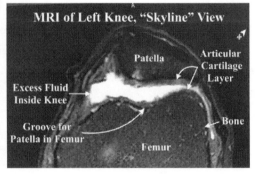

CT scans show more soft tissue detail and certain other abnormalities than x-ray but less than MRI. They are mostly useful in evaluating fractures where they can help in deciding the need for surgery as well as the best approach for reconstructing the fracture.

Bone scans are performed by injecting a short-lived, radioactive material into a patient's veins. This material is preferentially incorporated into bone-forming cells, following which a scanner is used to demonstrate areas of higher-than-normal incorporation. Such processes as fracture healing, infection, and cancer generate the appearance of "hot spots" to point the diagnostician to areas of abnormality for more detailed evaluation. The exposure to radioactivity is reportedly low, no more than one would get from a routine chest x-ray.

Synovial Fluid Analysis
Fluid is secreted into the joint by synovium (the joint lining). Usually, it is a thin, oily fluid with just enough volume to keep the inner surfaces of the joint slippery. Injury, infections, and certain kinds of arthritis cause an increase in the fluid, resulting in what is called an "effusion". Consider a deflated balloon with a drop of oil inside. The surfaces rub together with almost no resistance, and the balloon remains very flexible. Then fill the balloon with water and it becomes tighter and more rigid as more is added. A joint with excess fluid loses some of its range of motion, and if it becomes tense with fluid, it becomes stiff and can be excruciatingly painful.

When synovial fluid aspirated (removed with a needle) from a joint is analyzed, the process is called "synovianalysis".

Blood: Bloody fluid is consistent with injury to structures that have a robust blood supply. One is most likely to see this with tears of the ACL or PCL and with fractures extending into the joint. Although microscopic amounts of blood may be found, gross bleeding does not usually appear with meniscal tears since menisci have minimal blood supply.

Crystals: Gout and pseudogout are types of arthritis that can be diagnosed by synovianalysis. Polarizing microscopes can inform us if the crystals rotate light to the right or left, a key to distinguishing one crystal from the other.

Infection: If a joint is infected, it will likely appear cloudy and have a very high white blood cell count, generally multiple times higher than the white cell count in one's blood taken from a vein. Keep in mind it is essential to identify the organism before starting antibiotics, so DO NOT START YOURSELF ON ANTIBIOTICS BEFORE JOINT FLUID HAS BEEN COLLECTED. Aspirating the joint and doing cultures and other tests in a laboratory are done for that purpose. Broad-spectrum antibiotics (those that cover a variety of suspected bacteria) are started. Once cultures have identified the offending organism (usually within 48 hours, but sometimes after several days), the antibiotics can be changed to specifically target those bacteria. If a swollen joint is red and hot and the joint fluid is cloudy, it is probably a bacterial infection. Some organisms, such as TB (tuberculosis) and fungi, however, can cause the joint to be swollen and the fluid cloudy, but with no redness or heat. We have to keep our minds open to numerous possibilities.

Blood Studies (from Veins)

White Blood Cells: In infection, the white cell count is typically highly elevated with a predominance of a certain type of white cells. They can be elevated for other reasons, however, and some infections do not cause much elevation of the white cell count.

Erythrocyte Sedimentation Rate, (Sed rate, ESR) is an old but useful test. Blood is placed in a vertical, transparent tube. The time it takes for red cells to settle ("sediment") due to gravity is measured. The faster the rate of sedimentation, the higher the ESR. Finding a high ESR is similar to finding a high temperature; it is indicative of an inflammatory disorder in the body, but specific to no particular one. Not only is it a sign of current inflammation, but also measuring it over days or weeks can help your physician determine the course of the disease process.

CRP (C-Reactive Protein): Manufactured in the liver, CRP levels increase with inflammation. Like the ESR and body temperature, it is non-specific but can be helpful in determining the presence of infection and in evaluating a patient's progress with an inflammatory process, such as infection, certain types of arthritis, and cancer.

Arthritis Tests: Rheumatoid factor is present in 80% of adults with rheumatoid arthritis. A positive antinuclear antibody (ANA) test is an indicator of autoimmune disorders such as systemic lupus erythematosis (SLE), another type of inflammatory arthritis. Presence of Human Leukocyte Antigen B27 (HLA-B27) in your blood is not diagnostic for this disease, but its presence indicates a predisposition for ankylosing spondylitis, a type of inflammatory arthritis that mainly affects the spine and, to a lesser extent, the shoulders and hips.

Uric Acid: Elevated levels of uric acid in the blood are sometimes found during attacks of gouty arthritis.

Body Temperature
Measuring your body temperature with a thermometer seems so mundane it would be easy to overlook. Elevations of body

temperature, of course, are indicative of inflammation in the body. Like the ESR and CRP, it is non-specific, but very useful.

Chapter 5
Treatment of Knee Pain

The All Important Quadriceps Muscle Group

If you want to walk and if you want to have a strong knee, you must have strong quadriceps femoris muscles (the "quads"). This is the group of four muscles that straighten the knee, keep you from falling, help you arise from a chair, and guide the patella in its groove. We agree with the gerontologist who said that this is the muscle that keeps you out of a wheel chair. Almost all knee treatments require good quadriceps strength to make them successful; so a determined effort to achieve the best possible quad power is essential.

Quad strengthening is easy to understand, but to be successful you must be diligent and committed. One way is to sit on the side of a table or bed and straighten the knee with a small amount of weight attached to your foot or ankle. Straighten it as far as you can while contracting the quad as vigorously as you can. Focus on rigidly tightening the muscle once the knee is fully straight. Then lower it slowly. In doing so you employ three different kinds of therapy. First, you are doing "isokinetic exercise" which is strengthening while moving the joint. Next, when you are tightening the muscle once the knee is fully extended, you are doing "isometric exercise", strengthening therapy without moving the joint. Finally, when you slowly lower the foot, you are performing a "negative exercise", resisting movement while the muscle is lengthening, as opposed to shortening. We suggest doing sets of ten of these exercises at least daily. Lift the leg slowly, then hold it as straight and as hard as you can for six seconds; then slowly let it go back down.

If you want to really work your quads, you can do isometric exercises almost anytime, anywhere. When standing or lying, straighten the knee by tightening the quad as much as you can and hold it there for six seconds. Relax and repeat. Do this in sets of 10 or just do it as often as you think of it. You can even do it in secret when you are in a boring conversation at a social event while smiling inside, knowing you are accomplishing something of value at the time.

Internal Derangement

As you will remember from Dave's knee history, he suffered a meniscus tear when in college and had surgery about 10 years later. In his fifties, he had repeat surgery, this time with the arthroscope. It helped.

The term "internal derangement" is a non-specific term used to allow the doctor to keep an open mind about what may be wrong in a patient's knee, especially if it is not clearly arthritic. The usual offenders are tears of the menisci and loose bodies. In both situations the symptoms are pain, "giving way" while walking on level ground, and "locking", meaning that the knee gets stuck in a bent position. It will not fully straighten, and it hurts to bear weight.

With MRI, your surgeon can usually diagnose what is wrong and recommend what to do. Typically the treatment is arthroscopic surgery to remove the loose body or the torn portions of the meniscus. Dave's second surgery was to remove a torn lateral meniscus; the medial meniscus had already been removed. It helped prevent the locking and giving way that he had been having, but his knee was far from being restored to normal. On the other hand, he remained able to stand for long periods and was not subject to having the knee buckle unexpectedly.

Arthroscopy for arthritis has justifiably gotten a bad reputation in the treatment of arthritis. This will be addressed in detail in the section on arthritis.

Bursitis

Many joints have bursae, small sacs that lie between tendons and bones, over which the tendons glide. Bursae have very smooth inner walls and reduce friction with motion. There are many bursae around the knee, but the one that usually causes trouble is the pes anserine bursa that resides between a convergence of three tendons and the medial aspect of the upper tibia. When this becomes inflamed, the pain is felt just below the medial joint line. Non-steroidal-anti-inflammatory medications ("NSAIDs" such as ibuprofen and naproxen), local application of heat, a neoprene knee brace, and occasional injections of cortisone are standard treatments. We have never seen or heard of surgery being required. Pain occurring below a joint can originate from the joint. Likewise, pain in the pes anserine bursa area can be referred from the inside of the knee joint, such as from a degenerative or torn medial meniscus. If the tenderness is well below the knee joint and not at the joint line, it is probably bursitis. If the tenderness is not that localized and symptoms persist, MRI may be needed for a definitive diagnosis.

Baker's Cyst (also known as a "popliteal cyst"): Twenty percent of people are born with a small channel that connects the inside of their knees to a bursa sac in the back of the knee (the popliteal space). When these adults develop an "effusion" (excess fluid in the joint), this is typically due to a torn cartilage or arthritis. Fluid from inside the knee can migrate into and fill the bursa in the back of the knee. Sometimes the cyst is as bothersome as the abnormality inside the knee. It can be treated by removing fluid and injecting cortisone. On rare occasions, surgical removal is indicated, but in most cases your surgeon will elect to treat the problem inside the knee and ignore the "cyst", since it will usually subside on its own.

So, remember Richard, the fellow with the Baker's Cyst discussed in Chapter 3? We recommended an MRI of his knee and calf to further evaluate both the joint and the cyst. We expect he will have arthroscopic medial meniscectomy, and the cyst will subside on its own. That is up to him, of course. He may try having the fluid aspirated with a needle and injecting the cyst with cortisone. That will not cure anything but could allow him to defer knee surgery.

Tendonitis

Tendonitis is the result of micro-tears in tendons. Very active seniors may suffer tendonitis from tears in the patellar tendon below or the quadriceps tendon above the patella. Patellar tendonitis is felt in the tendon between the patella and its attachment to the tibia. It is especially painful with walking up stairs, running, and jumping. Pain from an arthritic patella is often felt below the patella, however, so it is important to distinguish one from the other.

Treatments include NSAIDs, heat, and a patella strap that goes around the knee just below the patella. We advise against cortisone injection, which could increase the likelihood of rupture of the tendon. Surgery is avoided if at all possible since, given enough time, the tendonitis usually subsides.

Quadriceps tendonitis occurs in the tendon attaching the quadriceps muscles to the patella. If this tendon ruptures, you will lose your ability to actively straighten your knee. If you find you are having pain just above the patella, be careful about stepping or jumping down from a height, as this is the kind of activity that could cause rupture. If it continues to hurt with walking up stairs, or especially with walking on level ground, you should seek help. Hopefully, avoidance of painful activities or even a protective brace for six to eight weeks will allow it to heal. If a complete tear occurs, you will need surgery to be able to use your quad thereafter.

We have not diagnosed tendonitis of the hamstring tendons. Hamstring problems are typically in the muscle itself where one can get a "hammie" or "hamstring pull" in the back of the thigh. These typically heal spontaneously with no surgery required. Unfortunately they can be very painful and typically require at least six weeks to heal. During that time you can do some gentle stretching to avoid losing the ability to fully straighten your knee, but you should avoid strenuous activities such as running and playing tennis. A compression sleeve around the thigh may make it feel better, but it can also give you a false sense of security and does not accelerate healing. Basically, you must give it time to heal. Do not keep testing to see if healing has occurred. Every time you stress and make it hurt, you can expect healing to take an additional six weeks.

Instability
When ligaments are torn, you can develop wobbling and slipping of the knee bones. Everyone has heard about tears of the ACL (anterior cruciate ligament), a sports injury seen in high performance athletes who must stop and start, twist and turn, and jump and land quickly. In younger athletes, the ACL is essential. Seniors, however, are less likely to be involved in such sports, and joints tend to stiffen with age. Repair of the ACL by sewing it back together does not work. Reconstruction using a graft from one's body or a cadaver is the usual surgical treatment. Considerable recovery and rehabilitation time is required, however, so we recommend very careful consideration of the potential benefits and the extensive rehabilitation

necessary before having it performed. A good muscle strengthening program and a stabilizing brace for sports such as tennis suffice in most cases.

Tears of the PCL (posterior cruciate ligament) are even less likely to need surgical treatment in seniors. Muscle strengthening should suffice. A brace for sports could also be necessary.

The MCL (medial collateral ligament) and LCL (lateral collateral ligament) keep the knee from sagging inward (valgus) and outward (varus). Quad strengthening and sometimes bracing for sports should be sufficient for tears in seniors.

Malalignment

The normal knee is aligned in a few degrees of valgus (an angle where the apex is medial). Due to a wider pelvis, women normally have a few degrees more valgus than men. Some people, however, are born with a propensity to be "knock kneed" or "bowlegged", a

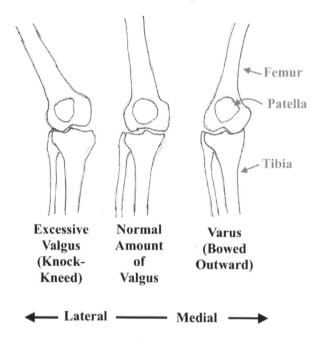

**Alignment
Frontal View of the Right Knee**

Femur

Patella

Tibia

Excessive
Valgus
(Knock-
Kneed)

Normal
Amount
of
Valgus

Varus
(Bowed
Outward)

◄— Lateral —— Medial —►

result of malalignment between the femur and tibia. In those cases, the pressure on the joint surfaces is not applied evenly. Some parts get too much pressure causing them to wear more than they should. Realignment is commonly done in younger people, especially if they are having pain that can be attributed to improper alignment. This is a big deal, however, as it requires cutting through the bone, realigning it, and then stabilizing it with fixation devices until the bones unite. Seniors, however, are already on the road to total knee replacement, which can also realign the joint. Furthermore, malalignment in seniors, such as seen in the above illustration, can be due to arthritis, which allows the joint space to narrow on one side and the knee to sag in the opposite direction. Thus, osteotomy (surgical cutting of the bone to realign it) alone would correct only part of the problem. We do not recommend it. In rare cases, realignment by osteotomy may be necessary to make total joint replacement successful, but that is indeed rare.

Malalignment of the extensor mechanism (the quadriceps muscles, the quadriceps tendon, the patella, and the patellar tendon) is fairly common, more so in women than men. This is mostly because women naturally have more valgus alignment (inward bowing) of their knees putting the patella at risk of riding up and down more laterally in the patellar groove. Sometimes the patella will sublux (slip partly out of place) and sometimes it will dislocate (slip completely out of place).

Here, again, the quadriceps muscles are very important. Some fibers of one of those muscles affect how the patella tracks through its groove in the femur. We recommend strengthening by starting with the knee in 15° – 20° of flexion (i.e. slightly bent) and straightening against light weights or just gravity. Moving it up and down from a 90° angle grinds away at the kneecap and is often unnecessarily painful. Isometric exercises, as described at the beginning of this chapter, are also useful, and painless. For patellar tracking, one should do isometric exercises with the knee straight, as this is a painless way to strengthen the oblique fibers of the vastus medialis, the part of the quads that helps keep the patella in place.

Synovitis

Some disorders, such as rheumatoid arthritis, cause an extraordinary thickening of the synovium, the normally thin lining of joints. If this cannot be controlled by medications and if the thickening and fluid from synovitis (inflamed synovium) become too problematic, the synovium may have to be removed. This can be done with an arthroscope or with open surgery. Most commonly, when needed and especially in seniors, it is done as part of a total knee replacement operation.

Arthritis

Dave had one injury and two subsequent operations on his knee. The operations bought him time, but his knee ultimately failed. Again, he had to do something. As we have discussed, surgeons basically consider two kinds of treatment: conservative, which means non-operative, and surgery. For arthritis, one should start with conservative treatment.

Conservative Treatment for Arthritis

The first step is over-the-counter (OTC) medications, typically NSAIDs such as ibuprofen, naproxen, and others. Acetaminophen can be very helpful, too, even though it is not an NSAID. Many people do well for years with such treatment.

If OTCs are not strong enough, your physician can prescribe stronger ones. This can further extend the period where nothing more needs to be done. Unfortunately, all drugs have side effects, so you must moderate your drug intake and monitor for potential problems, such as intestinal bleeding and kidney and liver damage.

Oral NSAIDs are for all kinds of arthritis including osteoarthritis and degenerative arthritis. Topical forms of NSAIDs can be applied to the skin over a painful joint or tendon. Colchicine is a specific drug for the symptoms of gout and may be helpful for pseudogout. Allopurinol can lower the levels of uric acid in your blood resulting in fewer attacks of gout. Rheumatoid arthritis, psoriatic arthritis, and others in the autoimmune category can be treated with immune therapy, both by IV (intravenous infusion) and orally.

You should also consider lifestyle changes. Instead of running, try bicycling, using an elliptical machine, or swimming to exercise. Among the worst things you can do to your knees is to gain weight. **Do not give up exercise and become obese.** If you are obese, losing weight can really help.

Cortisone is the next step. An <u>injection</u> into the knee can give significant and prompt relief, but the duration of relief is generally only for a few weeks or months. As with almost everything good in medical treatments, there are potentially bad side effects. No matter how carefully your provider does the injection, there is always a chance of introducing infection from the outside. Then you have an additional and possibly more difficult problem. Furthermore, excessive cortisone injections can accelerate the deterioration of the joint. We recommend injections no more often than three times per year in any one joint.

Cortisone type pills and injections into muscle or veins are used during severe inflammatory episodes. The potential side effects of bone loss leading to osteoporosis, damage of the blood supply to bones like the head of the femur at the hip, fluid retention, and intestinal bleeding, however, make the long term use of these medications undesirable.

Biologic Treatments

Hyaluronic acid is a natural part of joint fluid and formulations of it are available for injection into joints. We consider it "biologic oil". Depending on the product and your physician, you can have it all in a single dose or in a series of doses. The main concerns are infection and allergy. Since many hyaluronic acid products are extracts from rooster combs, people with chicken allergies are at risk. Fortunately, there are other products that do not come from chickens. Only about 50% of people get any benefit from these injections and the duration of improvement is variable. Those whose x-rays demonstrate "bone-on-bone" contact are unlikely to get any relief.

Orthobiologics / "Regenerative Medicine": Stem cells and PRP (platelet rich plasma) are in high demand as patients and physicians continue to seek breakthroughs in treatment for arthritis. In these treatments, blood, fat or liquid bone marrow is taken from the patient, filtered and spun in a centrifuge to concentrate beneficial stem cells. Specific layers are collected in a syringe and injected into patients' tendons to encourage healing of micro-tears and into arthritic joints to reverse inflammation and degenerative changes.

Meredith, a 71-year-old, active grandmother, stopped walking and playing golf because of severe knee pain. She had short-term relief from NSAIDs and injections of cortisone. Her imaging studies showed extensive degenerative arthritis with torn menisci. Two orthopedic surgeons recommended knee replacement. She decided to try injections of PRP, bone marrow and fat cells. After a few months her knee pain resolved. She has returned to golf and is able to walk long distances.

Testimonials and anecdotal reports are encouraging, and we are optimistic, but supportive scientific data are lacking. Following is a quote from an article in an American Academy of Orthopaedic Surgeons (AAOS) publication about stem cell treatments for arthritis: "Consequently, clinical use of these treatments has greatly outpaced evidence-based research." (Please see https://www.aaos.org/CustomTemplates/Content.aspx?id=6442 463013.). We applaud efforts to find less invasive ways to treat joint pain and tendonitis and look forward to seeing proof of efficacy in the future. Biologic treatments are expensive and are not covered by Medicare or most health insurers.

Alternative Treatments
There are many highly publicized homeopathic treatments for arthritis, most of which have not been proven beneficial.

Acupuncture is praised throughout the world as a treatment for many conditions. It is not within the expertise of the authors to say if it works, but we see no harm in giving it a try. Be sure the acupuncturist does not insert a needle into the joint itself as that could cause an infection. The knee joint capsule extends a couple of fingerbreadths above the patella, so make sure they do not place a needle too close to the upper aspect of the patella.

Herbs seem to work for some people. If they work for you, that is wonderful. Be aware that some herbs can interfere with certain medications such as anticoagulants like Coumadin and others. If you take prescription medications, consult with your physician or pharmacist before using herbal medications. That goes for what you rub on your skin as well as what you swallow. Many substances are absorbed through the skin, so it is possible to have negative side effects from topical applications.

WD-40 is a general-purpose lubricant that has been used by many for treatment of arthritis symptoms. Unfortunately, it is absorbed through the skin and has the potential to cause liver damage.

Burning: We once had a patient from a middle eastern country who had had his knee arthritis treated by placing the burning end of a stick against the skin in spots around the knees. When we saw him there were large round scars, but the skin was viable. He had terrible arthritis. The burning did not work, but total knee replacements made him happy.

Surgery for Arthritis

Deciding whether to have elective surgery

No matter how bad the pain, arthritis and tendonitis do not threaten your life. It is reasonable to tolerate the symptoms rather than have major surgery. Because only you can determine the severity of your pain and impairment, only you can make that decision.

When discussing surgery with our patients, we explained what to expect in the short and long terms and the potential consequences. When decision time came, we asked for a definitive answer from the patient. "Yes", meant yes, proceed with surgery. "No", meant no, and "maybe" also meant no. For those who were not sure they were ready to proceed, we advised them to wait until they were unequivocally ready.

It is rarely "too late" to get better, so there is generally no reason to "rush" into elective surgery.

Arthroscopic Surgery for people with arthritic knees has been done for years, but the results are not very good. Trimming frayed articular cartilage and punching holes in exposed bone to treat damaged joints in younger people may help them, but it is unlikely to help seniors. On the other hand, arthroscopic surgery may help seniors who have loose bodies or frayed and torn menisci that are getting jammed between bones and causing locking and giving way. Removing these loose objects does nothing for the arthritis, but it can help prevent giving way and falling. Although done through very small incisions, this is still major surgery that causes bleeding, swelling, and pain, so one should not assume it is anything less than a serious operation. Only if the problem is mechanical instability and not the aching pain of arthritis, is it worth a try.

In the following image taken at arthroscopy, you can see a frayed and torn medial meniscus. You also see areas of bare bone on the femur and tibia. Removing the torn meniscus in this case is unlikely to do much for the patient, and we cannot replace the joint surfaces through arthroscopic surgery.

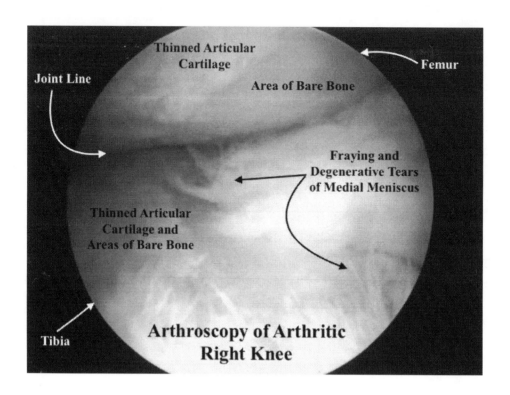

Arthroscopy of Arthritic Right Knee

Osteotomy is a surgical procedure where the bone is cut near, but not into, the joint, so the limb can be realigned. In those who are severely bowlegged or knock kneed, it might lessen the symptoms of arthritis in younger people. In seniors with arthritis, however, it is a big operation that is unlikely to provide enough relief to be worth going through.

Fusion of the bones together (arthrodesis) is a surgical procedure where the ends of the femur and tibia are removed, and then those bone ends are held tightly together until they unite. In essence, we are tricking the body into responding as if a fracture has occurred, initiating the same process as fracture healing. This can provide excellent pain relief, but the inconvenience of never again being able to bend the knee has made it unpopular as a treatment. In the face of an infected artificial joint, however, it may be the only way to cure the infection and allow for a functional leg.

Total Knee Replacement

Forty-five years after his knee injury, Dave's knee had badly deteriorated. It hurt so bad to walk that when he played golf, he rode a cart everywhere and did not walk around on the green to read putts. When he stood for long periods, the knee would feel stuck in place. His knee was beginning to bow outward. X-rays showed "bone on bone" (complete loss of the joint cartilage space). His orthopaedic surgeon recommended total knee replacement. Dave agreed. His surgery went well and he worked hard to rehabilitate. He became able to walk the golf course with ease and it even improved his game to the point he shot his age a

couple of times. He can almost fully straighten and bend his knee. He has some difficulty in walking down stairs. Walking up is no problem.

To say one is having a "total knee replacement" (TKR) is an oversimplification. As you have seen in the chapter on anatomy of the knee, it is composed of bones, articular cartilage, menisci, and ligaments, and is powered by large muscles. When the surgeon performs a TKR, he is only replacing

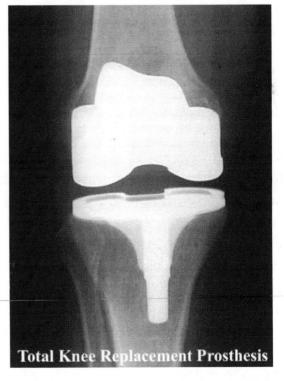

Total Knee Replacement Prosthesis

the surface of the bones with metal and plastic parts. You still need ligaments to hold the bones together and muscles to stabilize the joint and move the knee back and forth. During the process, the cuts in the ends of the femur and tibia are made so as to correct angular deformities at the time of replacement.

As there are three separate joint surfaces (those on the femur, tibia, and patella), three separate artificial components are inserted.

Femoral Component: The femoral component fits like a cap over the end of the femur. It is designed to mimic the normal end of the femur so that the artificial tibial component has a relatively natural shape to work against. In the front of this component, as in the front of the normal knee, there is a shallow groove that the patella glides through when the knee is flexed and extended.

Tibial Component: The mostly flat tibial component sits on the upper end of the tibia. There are shallow depressions on top of each side that match the convex ends of the femur. Depending on the condition of the knee before surgery, components with elevations in the middle of the tibial component can be selected to compensate for loss of one or both cruciate ligaments. Generally, a metal plate is attached to the top of the tibia and a plastic component is locked onto the plate. By waiting to insert the plastic part of the tibial component last, the surgeon can try test components of different thicknesses to adjust for stability and range of motion before inserting the permanent one.

Patellar Component: A dome-shaped patellar component is attached to the backside of the patella. Patellar components are made of plastic.

Attachment to Bone: The attachment of the prosthesis to bone is done with bone cement (methyl methacrylate). This acts as grout that works its way into the interstices of the bone ends and fastens the prosthetic components to the patient's bone. Loosening can occur, but that is only in a very low percentage of patients. An option is to have a roughened coating on the back of the prosthesis, permitting bone to grow into its interstices. That sounds good and works well in hips, but not as well in knees; knee prostheses are usually cemented into place.

Selection of Prosthesis: The orthopaedic manufacturing business is huge, and the competition among companies is fierce. As in other fields of medicine, advertising to the public is common. Fortunately, there are numerous excellent brands of prostheses, and the U. S. Federal Food & Drug Administration (FDA) has stringent requirements for implants (devices inserted into the body). Advertising a certain brand on television or promotion by a celebrity does not make it better than multiple other choices. **We recommend you select a surgeon you can trust and let your surgeon determine the type of prosthesis that works best in his or her hands.**

The same advice applies to custom-made prostheses. CT scans of your knee can be used to design a prosthesis just for you. Whether that actually works better than a standard prosthesis has yet to be proven. In every knee replacement there are four different components to be implanted (femoral, tibial tray, tibial insert, and patellar component). Your surgeon will have seven or eight sizes of each component from which to choose. This provides over 2,000 possible combinations of sizes. With preoperative planning, accurate "custom fitting" of the prosthesis to your knee can be achieved.

Type of Incision: "Minimal Incision Surgery" (MIS) is popular and laudable. The idea is to make incisions in the skin, tendon and muscle as small as possible to reduce pain and bleeding and to keep rehabilitation time to a minimum. On the other hand, a few inches of incision more or less has not been shown to improve the long-term results. The important consideration is for the incision to be large enough to allow your surgeon to do the best job possible.

Computer Assisted Surgery: Computer Assisted Total Knee Replacement (CATKR) can help the surgeon make precise bone cuts to correct knee deformities and align the knee. It works well, but it can add significant time to the operation. Experienced joint replacement surgeons can make precise bone cuts without CATKR. Many feel that the potential benefits in their hands are not worth the additional exposure time (the time the inside of your joint is exposed during surgery). **The longer the exposure time, the greater one's risk of infection and bleeding**.

Partial Joint Replacement

In some cases, it makes sense to replace only part of the knee joint. There are three distinct areas that, even though they are all in one large pouch, are called "compartments": patello-femoral compartment, medial compartment, and lateral compartment. If only one or two compartments are damaged, the surgeon may recommend replacing only one or two. The benefits of a partial joint replacement are it is reputed to feel more natural than a "total" and it can potentially "buy you time" before you need a TKR. Although it is appealing, it is still a major operation. It may make sense if you are age 50, but if you are 70, you may want to consider having the definitive procedure rather than planning to have another in 10 or 20 years.

What can you do to help yourself in advance of surgery?

Consult with your primary care physician to be sure you do not have anything that needs to be treated or corrected before surgery. Do not wait until the last minute.

Build strength in your muscles, especially those all-important quads. It is a lot easier to do so before you have a sore knee than afterwards, and it works better, too.

What can you do to help yourself after you have recovered from surgery?

Avoid running and jumping as well as sudden starts and stops. These activities can cause loosening of the prosthesis and wear the plastic portion of the joint.

Maintain good oral hygiene, focusing on your teeth and gums. Medications can cause dry mouth with a lack of saliva. Use an over-the-counter, sugar-free saliva substitute to help prevent decay and gum disease.

Notify your primary care physician if you have signs of infection anywhere in your body, and get it treated promptly. There is urgency in preventing bacteria from spreading through your blood stream to the site of your artificial joint.

Do not put yourself at risk. Avoid falls, especially from heights. Stay off ladders and countertops. Wear stable and secure shoes that are easy to put on. Use walking aids such as a cane, walking stick, or walker, if necessary. Fractures around artificial joints are very challenging and will likely permanently diminish the functionality of the new joint.

Work at regaining a normal gait. Strengthen your muscles. Watch yourself in a mirror or store window while walking, and ask friends and family to tell when you limp. Using a cane until you can walk without limping can help you relearn a normal gait rather than learn to walk with a chronic limp.

Infection Prevention

Have all **dental work** (cavities, gum disease, broken or loose teeth, and cleaning) treated well in advance. Bacteria from dental diseases or procedures can enter the blood stream and cause infection around your new joint. It is a good idea to take antibiotics prior to dental work to protect your joint replacement from release of these oral bacteria into your blood stream. Although not all agree, we suggest you ask your surgeon or dentist to provide you with an antibiotic prescription to take before dental procedures, including cleaning.

Be sure your hospital checks for potentially serious **bacteria in your system**. A nasal swab can be used to check for MRSA (methicillin resistant staphylococcus aureus), which can cause joint infections. Other sources of infection, such as urinary tract infection, should be discovered and cured well in advance of surgery. Make sure you do not have infections, cuts, or sores in your skin. If so, these must be resolved before proceeding.

Shower the night before and the morning of surgery with an antibacterial soap.

Fall Prevention

Prepare your living facilities for when you return home. Remove trip hazards such as throw rugs. Secure loose electrical cords, add grab bars to shower and toilet areas, and install toilet seat extensions.

Expectations

Dave was very happy with his knee. He was pain free and very functional. He could walk anywhere. He knew not to run or jump, as those activities could cause the prosthesis to loosen or the plastic to prematurely wear out. Mortar on a brick is a grout that is hard to remove. If you want it off, you chip away with hard tools. The cement holding your knee prosthesis to bone is also a grout. If you want to loosen it, jump up and down. The brake pads on your car are made of a softer-than-metal material that gets compressed between hard metal surfaces. If you drive like a teenager and often slam on the brakes, you can prematurely wear them out. Likewise, the plastic spacer in your artificial knee is a softer-than-metal material that gets compressed between metal surfaces. If you play sports that require you to rapidly start and stop, you can prematurely wear it out, too. Many surgeons allow their patients to play tennis. Dave elected golf.

When you awaken from the anesthesia of being put to sleep or sedation if you had spinal or nerve block anesthesia, you may be without pain. Surgeons now have long lasting local anesthetics they can inject into the tissues to prolong the effect. In addition, you may have prolonged nerve blocks to slow the onset of postoperative pain.

The next two or three days will likely be quite painful, however, so you will probably need strong pain medicines. After that, you should do your best to switch to OTC pain medications such as acetaminophen. You surgeon may instruct you to take aspirin as a partial anticoagulant to prevent DVT. If so, do it. If not, however, do not take aspirin or other NSAIDs, such as ibuprofen, since they could cause you to have excessive bleeding into your knee or elsewhere.

Ice packs and cooling machines can help avoid excessive swelling and reduce pain. Use them judiciously, of course, and be sure you follow the instructions of your surgeon in their use.

You will likely be allowed to bear weight as tolerated. At the beginning you will need a walker or crutches, but as your pain subsides and your quad strength returns, you will need less in the way of walking aids.

The first two weeks are critical in regaining your range of motion. Even though it hurts, you need to promptly straighten the knee and bend it past 90°. After a couple of weeks, the difficulty to bend markedly increases. By six weeks after surgery, you should have over 130° of flexion. A physical therapist is essential in this process, but the therapist cannot be with you all of the time. To be successful, you need to almost constantly work on maximum extension and flexion. We recommend that when lying down you elevate your leg with the foot on a pillow in such a way as to let gravity help you straighten the knee. If you cannot initially do this for long periods, do it for frequent short ones until you can go longer. Likewise, holding your knee in a position of the maximum flexion you can tolerate for periods of time can help you regain flexion. Another trick we recommend is to lie on your back with your fingers locked behind the thigh and bend the knee as much as possible. To push it even further, place the ankle of the non-operative leg over the ankle of the operative one and bear down to force more flexion.

Your therapist will encourage you to strengthen your quads as much as possible. Again, you have much more time to yourself to accomplish this. Lifting your entire leg off the bed is one good way to do it. In addition, whenever sitting or lying down, frequently tighten your quad as much as possible with your foot on a pillow. This not only helps strengthen the quad but it helps straighten the knee.

A home exercise bicycle can be helpful. Using a no-resistance setting and the bicycle seat raised as high as needed, rock the pedals back and forth until you can make a complete revolution. After you have done that a few times, lower the seat and do it again. Ultimately you can use this to work on range of motion and conditioning.

Be patient. People are not machines. Having a joint replacement is not like getting a new tire for your automobile and immediately speeding down the interstate highway. You can walk, but it will not be immediately normal. Rapid recovery is highly touted, but we typically warned our patients it took six weeks to start feeling good. After three months, you should have recovered about 80% with 90% recovery at six months and maximum medical improvement at about a year. You should be able to return to playing golf in six to twelve weeks.

That is the physical part. The mental effects are important, too. Many people fall into depression during the first week after surgery, just when they are seeing physical improvement. This often lasts for six weeks, and then goes away. We mention it to help you understand it is common and does not reflect on the patient in any way.

Revision Surgery
Hopefully, you will never need a revision, but we include it for completeness. The body constantly repairs itself, which is why our joints last as long as they do. Artificial parts, however, begin to wear immediately after being put to use. Fortunately, they usually outlast their hosts. Twenty or thirty years of satisfaction are not unusual, but if you get an artificial joint at an early age and live for a long time, you may outlast it. That is why we encourage people to wait as long as possible to get their joints replaced.

Some factors that accelerate the need for revision are loosening caused by infection or injury.

Revision of a total joint prosthesis is a significantly more extensive procedure than the initial replacement. As more exposure is needed and the scar from the original surgery is not as pliable as normal tissue, a longer incision will have to be made. Some or all of the original components have to be removed. There will also be reactive tissue in the joint that has to be removed. If the surface of a component has developed scratches, it needs to be replaced. Loose components are generally easier to remove, but if they are tightly adherent to bone, no matter how meticulous the surgeon, some bone will come out with the prosthesis. Swabs are taken to be sure there is no infection. If the tissues appear to be infected, your surgeon may insert temporary components until he is certain there is no infection. Typically this could mean waiting a week or two for the laboratory to be sure no bacteria have appeared in the culture dishes. If the joint is infected, the temporary prosthesis components will be left in place until the infection is cured.

Once everything is clean and ready, the surgeon can proceed. Bone grafts may be needed to make up for bone loss. Prosthetic components used in revisions usually have stems that go into the canals of the femur and tibia for extra stability.

Revision surgery is a big deal, *but it can be done and your chances of significant improvement are high.*

Chapter 6
Potential Complications of Knee Surgery

When we began telling preoperative patients about potential complications, some said their knee problems were so bad that surgery could not make them any worse. Unfortunately, that is wishful thinking; you need to know what could happen. The incidence of any of these complications is low, but the consequences are great. We take them seriously. Here are some you should know:

Infection: No matter how hard the surgical team tries, we cannot prevent infections every time. Treatment for an infected knee replacement involves aggressive antibiotic therapy and additional surgery. Since it is a foreign body, and foreign bodies make curing infection more difficult, the prosthesis usually has to be removed to allow eradication of the infection. Once the infection is gone, a new prosthesis can be inserted.

Skin Loss: The skin over the front of the knee is typically very thin and the blood supply can be poor. Incisions are planned to avoid skin damage. Nevertheless, a patch of skin over the front of the knee will occasionally die, leaving tendon exposed. If so, plastic surgery will be required to provide coverage with viable skin.

Metal Allergy: Most people with metal allergies are only allergic to nickel. The metals used in joint replacement are very low in nickel, and allergies to them are uncommon. "Rejection" of a prosthesis due to metal allergy is unusual. If a prosthesis were to be "rejected", your surgeon should check for a low grade infection as well as an allergy to the prosthesis.

Prosthesis Failure: The metal components of modern prostheses are very strong and rarely break. Ceramic components are used less often as they are more brittle, but the likelihood of their failing is low, too. The plastic tibial component is the part most likely to wear and break. If that happens, it will need to be replaced. Usually your surgeon can take out the old and snap in a new one. Keep in mind that this is a bigger operation than it may seem, so it is not to be considered lightly.

DVT (deep vein thrombosis), also known as "blood clots in the legs": DVT causes pain and swelling in the legs. Such a clot can break away from the vein wall and migrate into the heart to be pumped into the lungs (pulmonary embolus). This can cause serious breathing problems, even death. A permanent thrombus (clot that has turned into fibrous tissue) in a vein can cause chronic edema (swelling) of the extremity.

Nerve injury: Branches of the sciatic nerve run behind and around the knee. Any of these nerves can be damaged during replacement. Unique to the knee is a small branch of the saphenous nerve, the infrapatellar branch, which runs in the front of the knee just below the patella; it may be cut. That is not a complication of surgery; it is a consequence. The usual result is numbness and tingling on the front of the knee, mostly noticeably when kneeling.

Dave had a numb spot on the front of his knee. Like most people, it caused no pain or limitation and, after six months, he could kneel on the knee without difficulty.

On rare occasions patients will develop a painful neuroma (ball-shaped nerve ending) on the cut end of the nerve. If necessary, it can be treated with cortisone injections or surgically removed.

Vascular Injury: Along with the major nerves that run behind the knee are major blood vessels that are very close to the upper end of the tibia. It is possible to damage arteries and/or veins, as the bone cuts have to extend through the back of the tibia. If the injury is to a major artery or vein, it will have to be repaired; there is an increased likelihood of developing a DVT in a damaged vein. Most surgeons use a tourniquet cuff around the upper thigh to reduce bleeding during surgery. The pressure and time of use are carefully monitored. If the patient has arterial disease, use of a tourniquet could cause a problem with circulation in the leg.

Persistent Pain after Knee Replacement

Despite everything going well during and after surgery, some people keep hurting, and some develop pain months or years later. Here are some, but not all, potential causes:

Loose prosthesis: Knee prostheses are typically cemented into place, so early loosening is unusual. If early loosening occurs, one should consider infection. Given enough time, any of the components can loosen and become painful. Loosening may be obvious on x-ray, but not always. If symptoms persist, additional testing and even repeat surgery may be necessary to determine if the prosthesis is loose and needs to be replaced. If the prosthesis is obviously loose, it should be replaced to prevent further damage to the bone.

Infection: Highly virulent (aggressive) bacteria can cause obvious infection that becomes apparent soon after surgery. Bacteria with low virulence, however, can cause infections that are not obvious. Deep infection should be considered if there is greater than expected drainage following knee replacement, or if there was a "superficial infection" that required a course of antibiotics. Infection may cause loosening of the prosthesis. Treatment of deep infection involves removing the prosthesis and infected tissue to the extent possible and replacing the prosthesis. Our preference is to initially replace the prosthesis with temporary components, try to eradicate the infection with antibiotics, and then insert a new prosthesis once the infection has been cured. Some surgeons, however, advocate inserting the final prosthesis during what is called a one-stage procedure and then trying to cure the infection with antibiotics.

Tendonitis: Tendonitis is not usually a complication of knee replacement. On the other hand, the patellar tendon, the one that connects the patella to the tibia, is put under significant stress at the attachment on the tibia during joint replacement. It can be partially or completely torn during surgery. A partial tear could cause pain at the attachment site. A complete tear of course, would have to be repaired.

Referred pain: Hip pain is notorious for being sensed in the knee. If the pain is felt in the front of the thigh down to and including the knee and no other cause for persistent knee pain is found, one should evaluate the hip.

Caveat: *Despite what you have read in this chapter, the odds are overwhelming that you will have no serious complications, and you will do just fine.*

Glossary

Positions of Body Parts

Proximal and Distal: Relates to the location of one body part toward or away from another body part
>   **Proximal**: Closer to the trunk or body part in discussion
>>   Example: In the lower extremity, the knee is proximal to the ankle.
>   **Distal**: Further from the trunk or body part in discussion
>>   Example: In the lower extremity, the ankle is distal to the knee.

Frontal View of Knees

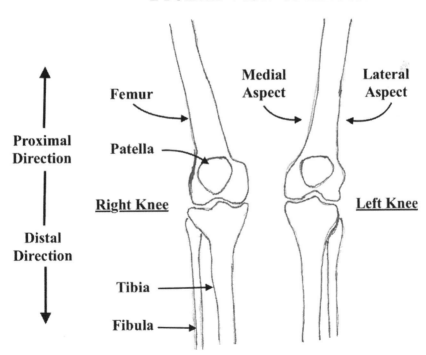

Medial and Lateral: Relates to the sagittal plane of the body (the plane that "divides" the body into right and left portions)

    Medial: Toward the middle of the body relative to some other body part

        Example: The naval is medial to the side of the body.

    Lateral: Away from the middle of the body

        Example: The side of the body is lateral to the naval.

**Alignment
Frontal View of the Right Knee**

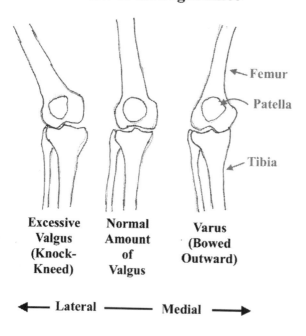

| Excessive Valgus (Knock-Kneed) | Normal Amount of Valgus | Varus (Bowed Outward) |

← Lateral —— Medial →

Alignment

    Varus: The angle of deformity (malalignment) points laterally. "Bowlegged" people have varus deformities at their knees.

    Valgus: The angle of deformity points medial. "Knock-kneed" people have valgus deformities at their knees.

Flexion and Extension

Flexion: The bending of an extremity or the spine at a joint or joints

> **Degrees of Flexion**: The "neutral position" of the knee (and other joints) is considered straight. When one is sitting in a chair with the feet on the floor the knees are in approximately 90° of flexion.

Extension: The opposite of flexion of an extremity or spine at a joint or joints.

> **Hyperextension**:   Passing beyond the neutral position and going into an overextended position
>
> > **Examples**
> >
> > When the knee is "bent backwards", it is hyperextended.
> >
> > When the wrist is bent backwards, it is hyperextended.
> >
> > When one leans backward beyond the usual erect position of the spine, the spine is in hyperextension.

Anterior and Posterior: Relates to the coronal plane of the body [the plane that "divides" the body into the front (ventral) and back (dorsal) portions]

> **Anterior**: Toward the front of the body relative to another part or parts
>
> > **Example**: The toes are anterior to the heel.
>
> **Posterior**:   Toward the back of the body relative to another part or parts
>
> > **Example**: The heel is posterior to the toes.

Tendons, Ligaments, and Bursae

Tendon: The continuation of a muscle that attaches muscle to bone

Muscles are attached to bone in at least two places, and these attachments are through a transition of the beefy muscle tissues into tendons. Tendons can be long and cable-like or so short that the beefy part of the muscle appears to be attached to bone. The tendon attachment to bone is an actual blending of the tendon tissue into the soft tissue inside the bone. This is analogous to steel mesh in concrete. Tendons attach above and below a joint so that when they contract, they move the joint. Muscles move joints by actively shortening (contracting). To allow a joint to move, they relax on the side opposite the side on which the muscles contract.   Muscles contract on the flexion side of a joint to bend it, and contract on the extension side to straighten it.

Ligament: Similar in structure to tendons, ligaments are the tough structures that hold bones together to make joints. Like tendons, ligaments can be a variety of lengths and shapes from wide like straps to round like cables. Also like tendons, the soft tendinous tissue blends into the bone attaching to the soft tissue within it.

Cruciate Ligaments: Round ligaments in the center of the knee that limit forward and backward movement of the tibia relative to the femur. The anterior cruciate ligament (ACL) limits forward movement of the tibia. The posterior cruciate ligament (PCL) limits backward movement of the tibia.

Medial Collateral Ligament (MCL): Strap-shaped thickening of the medial capsule that prevents excessive valgus instability (medial bending of the knee joint)

Lateral Collateral Ligament (LCL): Cable-shaped ligament stretching from the femur to the top of the fibula that prevents varus instability of the knee (bowing)

Bursa: Envision a plastic bag containing a thin layer of oil. Then move the surfaces of the bag back and forth over each other to sense the low resistance. Bursae are similar. They are pouches with smooth inner surfaces and contain oil provided by the body. They are found in areas where tendons and ligaments rub back and forth over bone, reducing friction at those spots. When normal, they are thin and flexible and assume the shape of the structures around them. When abnormal, they swell with fluid and become painful.

Arthritis

The word "arthritis" is derived from the root words "arthro" for joint and "itis" for inflammation. Although there are many types of arthritis, we will limit this section to those more commonly seen.

Osteoarthritis: Generalized arthritis affecting multiple joints. Excess bone is laid down and osteophytes (bone spurs) occur. A hallmark is that the bony parts of the joint become harder and the joint cartilage space narrows. Osteoarthritis is commonly attributed, but not limited, to the aging process.

Degenerative Arthritis: This diagnosis is generally applied to one or a few joints in absence of generalized arthritis such as found in osteoarthritis. Otherwise there is no apparent difference from osteoarthritis in function or in appearance at surgery or by x-ray. When arthritis follows injury such as fracture or other damage to the articular surface or cartilage, it is called "posttraumatic degenerative arthritis".

Inflammatory Arthritis: Thinking simply, osteoarthritis and degenerative arthritis are characterized by mechanical problems that result in a mild to moderate inflammatory response. Inflammatory arthritis, on the other hand, is characterized by inflammation that results in mechanical problems. In certain types of arthritis, this inflammation is caused by an attack against the body by one's own immune system. In cases such as rheumatoid arthritis, this "autoimmune" attack results in a marked proliferation of the synovium lining the joint and release of enzymes that damage articular cartilage. Bone density diminishes. Like most diseases, these can be mild and transient or severe and permanent. Rheumatoid arthritis, systemic lupus erythematosis, Reiter's Disease, Sjögren's syndrome, and psoriatic arthritis are examples of inflammatory arthritis.

Gout and Pseudogout: These are also inflammatory arthritis, but not the autoimmune type. Microscopic crystals deposited into synovium stimulate an inflammatory response resulting in pain, swelling, and variable levels of joint damage. Gout is known to be caused by a malfunction in the liver allowing an increase in uric acid (a chemical in the blood) and can generally be managed with medication to help lower the amount of uric acid in the blood stream. Pseudogout (officially called CPPD, calcium pyrophosphate deposition disease) is also a type of arthritis caused by the deposition of crystals into synovium. The basic cause is not clear, but the incidence appears to increase with age. Treatment of acute flare-ups is directed at controlling inflammation.

Injuries

Fracture: Broken bone

Simple fracture

The bone is broken into only two pieces, and
The skin is not broken.

Comminuted fracture: The bone is broken into more than two pieces. It could be three pieces or 3,000 pieces, but if it is more than two, it is comminuted.

Compound fracture / Open fracture: The skin is torn open, exposing broken bone(s) to the outside of the body.

Angulated fracture: The bone fragments are bent in relation to each other.

Displaced fracture: The bones at the fracture site are offset in relation to each other. It is common for displaced fractures to also be angulated.

Fragility fractures: Fractures that occur in those with fragile bones such as those with osteoporosis. These are typically fractures of the "hip" and "wrist" and "compression fractures" of the spine. Adults who suffer any of these fractures should be tested for osteoporosis.

Fracture Patterns

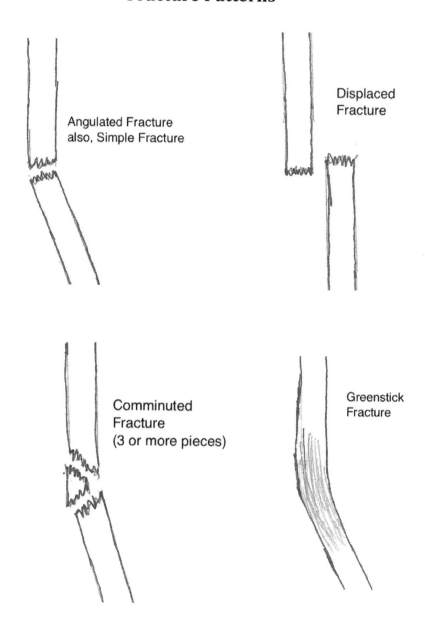

Angulated Fracture
also, Simple Fracture

Displaced
Fracture

Comminuted
Fracture
(3 or more pieces)

Greenstick
Fracture

Dislocation and Subluxation

Dislocation: The disruption of a joint where no part of a joint surface remains in contact with the opposite joint surface

The often-used phrase "complete dislocation" is redundant since the term dislocation means it is completely out of place.

Fracture-dislocation: A situation where the bones comprising the joint are broken as part of the injury resulting in dislocation

Thus, there is a fracture and a dislocation in the parts of the structures that make up the joint.

Subluxation: A partial disruption of a joint where some parts of the opposing joint surfaces remain in contact

> **Example**: When a shoulder "partially goes out", it is subluxed. [There is no such thing as a "partial dislocation". The joint is either dislocated or it is subluxed.]

Imaging Studies

MRI (magnetic resonance imaging): An image generated by a machine that uses powerful electromagnets to intermittently cause atoms in the body to misalign and then realign resulting in an emission of electromagnetic waves. MRI demonstrates both bone and soft tissues and helps find and define abnormalities.

CT Scan (CAT Scan, computerized axial tomography): Special computerized x-ray machines that provide much greater detail of bone and soft tissues than regular x-rays

Bone Scan: Imaging test that uses a radioactive substance injected into a subject's vein.   Bone is in a constant stage of turnover, which means that old bone is constantly being replaced by new bone. Cells making new bone preferentially incorporate this substance. If the bone is more active than normal, more of the substance will be taken up and a "hot spot" will appear on the image. The whole body is typically scanned making this a good study to use when looking for bone cancer and infection. Increased uptake is also seen during and long after fracture healing.

Diagnostic Ultrasound: Images can be created by bouncing sound waves off of soft tissues and bones. These studies require expert operators and can be performed quickly and inexpensively, but the images are not as distinct as those of MRI.

DVT Prevention

Anticoagulation
The phrase "blood thinning" is commonly used, but it is misleading. It suggests that you have diluted the blood, which would make the patient anemic without accomplishing the intent. In order to reduce undesirable clotting (coagulation) of blood, "anticoagulants" that interfere with blood clotting mechanisms are used. To prevent DVT (deep vein thrombosis) after surgery, physicians may partially anticoagulate their patients' blood for a few weeks. In some cases, patients need to be "fully anticoagulated".   Unfortunately, this puts them at greater risk of excessive bleeding from the surgical area and from minor injuries or lacerations.

Calf Pump

The heart pumps blood downhill under high pressure. Blood then passes through a bed of capillaries before flowing uphill to return to the heart. Imagine pumping a liquid downhill where it must squeeze through a sponge before returning to the pump several feet higher than the sponge. Also called the "second heart", the "calf pump" is an elegant mechanism. The veins below the knees have soft walls and run among the muscles of the calf. When those muscles tighten, they squeeze the veins forcing the blood to flow away. At the thigh level, veins have valves that direct the blood upward toward the heart. A result of malfunctioning valves is "varicose veins" that occur when the valves fail to keep blood from flowing backward (downhill) causing increased venous pressure. The veins dilate, become visible, and the legs swell.

Acknowledgements

We cannot sufficiently thank everyone who helped and inspired us along the way. Our wives have steadfastly stood beside us and in our places many times for many years. Without them, our careers as well as our lives outside of work would have been meaningless.

We owe a profound thanks to those who helped educate us: Our teachers in grammar school, high school, university, and medical school, and the professors in our orthopaedic training programs, all of whom gave so much of themselves to help us learn and understand our profession.

We deeply appreciate our volunteer readers who worked diligently to help make this book more readable and understandable: Linda Hundley, Marcie Brame, Kenneth Dickinson, Jack Kuske, Richard Keegan, and Chris and Richard Patterson. Any errors you find are ours, but without our readers there would be many more.

Finally, we greatly appreciate your reading this work. We would like to hear from you about what you like and do not like, so we can try to improve with each book. Posting a review on Amazon would be most appreciated.

Many thanks!

About the Authors

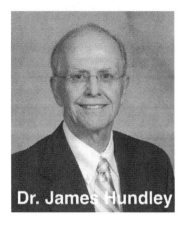

Dr. James Hundley

James D. Hundley, M.D. is a graduate of the University of the North Carolina School of Medicine and the Orthopaedic Surgery Residency Program of UNC Hospitals. After completing his training in orthopaedic surgery, he served as an orthopaedic surgeon in the U.S. Air Force for two years before joining an orthopaedic group practice in Wilmington, N.C.

His primary medical interests were in sports medicine where he was a division-one university athletic team physician for over twenty years and adult reconstruction (primarily hip and knee replacement surgery). Retired from medical practice, he continues to manage OrthopaedicLIST.com, a resource for orthopaedic surgeons founded in 2003.

Hundley's peers in orthopaedic surgery, the UNC School of Medicine, UNC-Wilmington, his community, and his state have recognized him for his efforts. He continues to serve on non-profit boards and a foundation focused on community health.

His writings include multiple scientific papers published in medical journals, numerous magazine articles, and two blogs: www.agingdocs.com and http://www.orthopaediclist.com/blog.

Hundley and his wife, to whom he has been happily married for over fifty years, have three children and five beautiful granddaughters.   His other interests include golf, fishing, and reading.

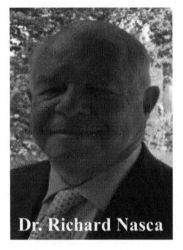

Dr. Richard Nasca

Richard J. Nasca, M.D. was born in Elmira NY and is a graduate of Georgetown College and Georgetown Medical School. He completed his internship at the Hospital of the University of Pennsylvania and postgraduate training in Surgery and Orthopaedics at Duke University and Affiliated Hospitals.

Dr. Nasca served as Chief of the Amputee and Hand Services at the Philadelphia Naval Hospital caring for Vietnam casualties.

Dr. Nasca held teaching appointments in Orthopaedic Surgery at the University of Arkansas School of Medicine and the University of Alabama School of Medicine. During his time in practice he specialized in caring for patients with spine deformities, injuries and disorders.

He has been married to Carol T. Smith, R.N. for fifty-two years and has three children and one granddaughter. Dr. Nasca lives in Wilmington N.C. He is a volunteer physician at local medical clinics, on Advisory Boards at the College of Health and Human Services at University of North Carolina at Wilmington and has published five books, several book chapters and seventy peer reviewed scientific articles.

Dr. Nasca works in the Good Shepherd Center soup kitchen and helps them raise funds, is a coach with the First Tee golf program for youths, and is a certified Master Gardener. He enjoys golf, gardening, swimming and travelling.

Reviewer Comments

This is "everything you always wanted to know about your knees"! After reading, MY KNEE HURTS!, I felt empowered with the language needed to describe my knee pain. Being able to adequately describe pain, will not only save time when meeting with the doctor, but also demystifies the medical terminology. Armed with this knowledge, I have a much greater understanding of my own situation.

--Marcie B.

Very readable book that takes the mystery out of knee anatomy while clearly describing knee problems and potential solutions.

--Chris and Rick, P.

My Knee Hurts *is very well written and important for me because I have experienced many of the situations that the book discusses. As I am planning for both of my knees to be replaced, I am now better prepared for my challenges. Dr. Hundley has given another wonderful gift to us aging Baby Boomers.*

--Rich K.

Having a knee problem? This book will be a valuable asset in helping you to understand what may be occurring in your knee, which is arguably the most complicated and necessary mechanism in your skeletal structure. You will be able to understand the test procedures your physician employs in developing a diagnosis in your case and will be able to share in the plan for your recovery.

--Jack K.

It is widely accepted that knowledge is the ultimate elixir. In this presentation, the doctors do not provide a guide to knee surgery; but they do provide a scenario that introduces a very worthy outline.

--Kenneth D.

Made in the USA
Middletown, DE
23 September 2018

 MAR 2019